Copyright ©

All rights reserved. No part of this publication maybe reproduced, distributed, or transmitted in any form or by any means, including photocopying, recording, or other electronic or mechanical methods, without the prior written permission of the publisher, except in the case of brief quotations embodied in critical reviews and certain other noncommercial uses permitted by copyright law.

Contents

What Is The Noom Diet?.................................7

How the Noom diet came to be 8

The Noom diet is safe to try for most 9

Is there any evidence for its effectiveness?.....10

    Research into the Noom app 11

How much does Noom cost? 13

So, will you lose weight on Noom? It can but you have to really commit. 13

How is Noom different than Weight Watchers (WW)? 16

How Does The Noom Diet works....................17

What does Noom actually do to help with weight loss?..18

What You Should Know 19

What Can You Eat? 22

Food to Eat 23

Food Not to Eat 24

Benefits.. 26

Drawbacks... 29

Is the Noom Diet a Healthy Choice for You? 31

Health Benefits... 32

Health Risks.. 34

Noom's food guide 35

Noom Diet Sample meal plan 36

Monday 37

Tuesday 37

Wednesday 38

Thursday 38

Friday 39

Saturday 39

Sunday 39

NOOM DIET RECIPES 40

Noom Green Meal 40

Egg Breakfast Cups 43

Coconut Energy Balls 45

Deconstructed Grilled Romaine Salad with Cherry Tomatoes, Charred Corn, and Avocado Cream Dressing 49

Healthy Slow Cooker Lentil and Vegetable Soup 53

Banana-Apple And Nut Oatmeal 55

Chicken And Avocado Pitta Pockets 57

Turkey Cheddar Tacos 59

Salsa Verde Chicken Tacos 61

Chinese Chicken Salad 62

Spicy Thai Basil Chicken 64

Chipotle Honey Mustard Chicken Fingers 66

Chicken Fajita Burritos 69

Brown Rice Chicken Risotto 72

Low-Calorie Chicken Tortilla Soup 74

Banana-Apple & Nut Oatmeal 78

Mini Ham and Cheese Quinoa Cups 79

Healthy Breakfast Sandwich 82

Apples and Cinnamon Breakfast Quinoa 85

Breakfast Jar Parfait 87

Green Monster Smoothie 90

FREEZER BREAKFAST SANDWICHES 91

Spinach Quiche Cups 93

Blueberry Flax Superfood Smoothie 97

Peanut Butter and Jelly Quinoa Egg Muffins 99

NO BAKE ENERGY BITES 103

Banana Cookie Overnight Oats 105

Ginger Banana Cookies 106

Party Potatoes.. 110

PROTEIN-PACKED OMELET 112

Avocado and Egg Lunch 114

Peanut Butter and Jelly Cottage Cheese Breakfast Bowl 116

What Is The Noom Diet?

The Noom weight loss program is not your typical diet plan. For instance, there are no off-limits foods or structured eating windows. Think of Noom as more of an all-around lifestyle shift that prioritizes healthy eating, regular exercise, stress management, and better sleep hygiene.

In fact, this popular weight loss program is psychologically driven. The basis for Noom's digital weight loss plan is cognitive behavioral therapy, a type of talk therapy used in clinical psychology settings.

Noom's wide-angled and long-term approach to health helps people shift their mindset and approach weight loss differently. Instead of focusing on quick results, Noom teaches people how to shift their perspectives about weight and understand the importance of physical activity and why good nutrition affects much more than the number on a scale.

Nutrition is an important component of the Noom weight loss program since a healthy, balanced diet is integral to long-term weight management. The Noom app is a helpful resource for tracking progress and provides ongoing support from certified health coaches. Noom uses a color-coded approach to nutrition: It labels foods as green, yellow, or red based on their nutrient density and how often you should eat them.

How the Noom diet came to be

The Noom app was created in 2008 by Saeju Jeong and Artem Petakov. According to the company website, the Noom diet was developed with an emphasis on psychology as much as nutrition.

It is not a prescribed diet in the sense that it doesn't restrict you to a certain type or amount of food. Rather it's a way to plan meals and change behavior with the support of a group.

The Noom diet is safe to try for most

The Noom diet is safe for anyone to try. Noom provides a minimum number of calories per day, encouraging people not to restrict food in an unsafe or unhealthy way.

It uses evidence-based behavior changes and smart coaches to help people set and achieve their weight goals.

Is there any evidence for its effectiveness?

Apps such as Noom encourage people to self-monitor their weight loss on a regular basis. A 2017 study found that people who frequently and consistently record their dietary habits experience more consistent and long-term weight loss.

However, self-monitoring weight loss is a practice that tends to decrease quickly over time. To prevent this, the Noom app provides features to motivate people to continue self-monitoring.

These features include access to both a health coach and a social platform where people can discuss their weight loss challenges and successes with other users.

Research into the Noom app

In 2016, some researchers conducted a study of the effectiveness of the Noom app. The study analyzed dietary data from Noom users who recorded what they ate at least twice a month for 6 months.

Of 35,921 Noom users, 77.9% reported a reduction in body weight while using the app. The researchers found that users who monitored their weight and dietary habits more frequently experienced more consistent weight loss.

In a separate study, also from 2016, researchers used Noom to deliver a diabetes prevention program (DPP) to 43 participants with prediabetes. At the start of the study, each participant had either overweight or obesity. The purpose of the study was to investigate the efficacy of the DPP in promoting weight loss among the participants.

The participants had experienced significant weight loss by week 16 and week 24 of using the DPP. Of the 36 participants who completed the study, 64% lost more than 5% of their body weight.

However, the study did not compare the Noom diet with any other app or diet. It is, therefore, difficult to know whether the Noom diet is any more effective than other weight loss strategies.

How much does Noom cost?

There is a free version, although Noom also has paid versions (it's about $59 a month, but you can buy multiple months at the same time for less money). In the paid version, you fill out a more detailed questionnaire about your lifestyle and health goals, plus what might be holding you back from achieving your weight-loss goals.

So, will you lose weight on Noom? It can but you have to really commit.

It's definitely possible, but it really comes down to whether you'll actually use it consistently.

According to a 2016 study in the journal Scientific Reports, Noom can help with weight loss. Researchers analyzed data from 35,921 Noom app users over the course of about nine months and found that 77.9 percent reported they lost weight. One interesting tidbit: Those who neglected recording their dinner in the app lost less weight than those who recorded their dinner regularly.

So while the app can definitely help you lose weight—you have to actually use it, as I mentioned. If you really take advantage of the app daily and put in data that's honest and truthful, the Noom program should help you lose weight. In other words, listen to the experts and follow the plan and you'll squash some goals.

The ideal user is probably someone with a busy lifestyle (hi, almost everyone on the planet!). And those who enjoy virtual support from like-minded peeps (shout-out to millennials) may also benefit.

Personally, I like that the app is realistic about long-term results and doesn't try to get its users to conform to a restrictive or fad-diet style of eating (e.g. keto, gluten free, raw, etc.).

Noom also helps users bring a sense of awareness to what they're eating throughout the day. That's usually the first step to sustained weight loss—focusing on what you're eating—without judgement or without labeling your eating habits "good" or "bad." Then, once you have a sense of awareness, you can tackle the reason you might be eating when you're not hungry, or why you turn to food out of stress, and then make any adjustments as needed.

How is Noom different than Weight Watchers (WW)?

The are similar in that they both use a food "ranking" system (with WW, it's a points system, whereas with Noom, it's a color system) to group foods as more and less nutritious. But Noom arguably gets more at the psychological factors behind weight management, and helps you explore why you have certain eating habits and choose the foods you do. WW, on the other hand, boasts a strong community that offers lots of accountability and external support. Noom is also a little bit pricier.

Which one is better for you? It ultimately depends on your personality and budget. Consider doing a consultation with a dietitian to help you choose, or ask friends and family who may have experience with the two programs.

How Does The Noom Diet works

Noom aims to help you lose weight like most commercial diet plans and programs — by creating a calorie deficit.

A calorie deficit occurs when you consistently consume fewer calories than you burn each day.

Noom estimates your daily calorie needs based on your gender, age, height, weight, and your answers to a series of lifestyle questions.

Depending on your goal weight and timeframe, Noom uses an algorithm to estimate how many calories you need to eat each day. This is known as your calorie budget.

For safety reasons and to ensure adequate nutrition, the app does not allow a daily calorie budget below 1,200 calories for women or 1,400 calories for men .

Noom encourages food logging and daily weigh-ins — two self-monitoring behaviors associated with weight loss and long-term weight loss maintenance.

What does Noom actually do to help with weight loss?

Any reduced-calorie diet plan or program can help you lose weight if you follow it.

Still, sticking with a diet is difficult for many people. Most diets fail because they're difficult to maintain.

To date, no studies have compared the effectiveness of Noom with other weight loss diets, but researchers have analyzed data from Noom users.

In one study in nearly 36,000 Noom users, 78% experienced weight loss while they were using the app for an average of 9 months, with 23% experiencing more than a 10% loss, compared with their starting weight.

The study also found that those who tracked their diet and weight more frequently were more successful in losing weight.

What You Should Know

Noom is not your typical fad diet, though some might think of Noom as a fad since it's a relatively new weight loss platform. But the difference is in the holistic approach—instead of promising rapid weight loss in just a couple of weeks or less, Noom guarantees lifelong weight management through renewed healthy habits.

At its core, Noom works like many digital weight loss programs. After you enter your information into the app, an algorithm builds a customized weight loss and fitness plan determined by your health status, demographics, goals, and more.

First, you'll choose whether you want to "get fit for good" or "lose weight for good." Then, Noom will direct you to a lifestyle quiz to help build your weight loss program. The Noom app requests the following information to build your plan:

- Demographics: Your age, current weight, height, and sex

- Goals: Your health goals—specifically how much weight you want to lose

- Lifestyle: A quiz to assess your work life, relationships, motivation to lose weight, and other factors such as your brain health, digestion, sleep, and energy levels

Once you're all set up, you'll get matched with a health coach and begin working toward your health goals. Through Noom's Healthy Weight Program, you'll have access to your assigned coach during normal business hours, as well as 24/7 access to a coach through the app's chat service. You'll use the Noom app for everything related to your weight loss plan including:

- Logging and tracking your food and portion sizes (by searching the Noom database or scanning barcodes)

- Tracking your water intake

- Logging and tracking your exercise

- Logging health metrics like your heart rate, blood pressure, and blood sugar

- Reading health articles and taking quizzes

- Communicating with your health coach and receiving one-to-one coaching during business hours

What Can You Eat?

The green-labeled foods on the Noom diet usually contain the most nutrients and least amount of calories, while red-labeled foods have more calories and fewer nutrients. Yellow-labeled foods fall somewhere in between. If you're unaccustomed to counting calories, tracking your daily caloric intake on the Noom diet plan may take some getting used to.

To track your food, you can search the Noom food database of more than 150,000 items, or scan supported barcodes on packaged foods. You can also log your food manually, which is helpful for those who like to cook homemade recipes.

Food to Eat

- Vegetables

- Fruits

- Meats

- Dairy products

- Whole grains

- Healthy fats

Food Not to Eat

- Processed foods

- High fat foods

- Added sugars

- Oils and condiments

The Noom diet does not specifically exclude any foods, which means the foods to avoid listed above don't have to be eliminated entirely. These red-labeled foods can still be consumed in moderation. The other food groups listed above include many options of what you can eat while on the Noom weight loss program as part of a healthy diet. The breakdown of green, yellow, and red label foods is as follows:

- Green label foods include nutritious vegetables like carrots, sweet potatoes, broccoli, and spinach. These, therefore, get the "green light" for the most consumption on the Noom diet. Fruits like apples, oranges, berries, bananas, and tomatoes, non-fat dairy items like yogurt, and whole grains like brown rice also fall into this category.

- Yellow label foods should be eaten "with caution" or less often than green label foods. These include lean proteins like grilled chicken, salmon, and turkey breast; low-fat dairy items including milk, cheeses, and eggs; healthy fats like avocado and olives; and grains and legumes such as beans, chickpeas, and quinoa.

- Red label foods are not completely off-limits but should be eaten with the least frequency. These include processed meats, some nut butters, oils and condiments, sugar, and high fat foods like pizza and french fries.

Benefits

Certified health coaches: All of Noom's health coaches go through a four-week training from Noom to become proficient in cognitive behavioral therapy, the method that drives Noom's weight loss program. However, not all Noom coaches are certified outside of the Noom training program (more on that under the cons below).

Psychological approach: Cognitive behavioral therapy is a proven psychological method that helps you understand the relationship between your feelings, thoughts, and behaviors.

Focus on the long-term: Because of Noom's psychological approach, the basis of the program lies in habit change, which is how you can lose weight for the long-term. Rather than inducing rapid weight loss for the first few weeks, Noom aims to help you develop a sustainable mindset around food, fitness, and wellness.

Focus on eating whole foods: With Noom, you won't ever have to buy frozen meals (unless you want to), premade shakes, or protein bars—the focus is eating healthy for life, which means selecting foods that satisfy both your tastebuds and your body. Noom's color approach (green, yellow, and red foods) helps you choose nutrient-dense foods without sacrificing your weight loss goals.

All-in-one support: Noom acts as your health coach, nutritionist, personal trainer, and accountability buddy all at the same time. If you're the kind of person who likes to minimize app clutter on your phone and prefers all of your health data in one place, Noom could be a great fit for you.

Scientifically supported: A number of scientific studies back up Noom's approach to weight loss (more on that below).

Drawbacks

Expensive: At a minimum of $59 per month, Noom costs more than many people may be willing or able to spend on a weight loss program

Language can be somewhat degrading: While Noom's user experience is designed to be motivating, it might feel derogatory to some people. For example, the app and website use language such as "conquer your food triggers," which is potentially problematic for those who genuinely struggle with food triggers or emotional eating.

No face-to-face option: If you thrive on face-to-face coaching, Noom might not be the right choice for you. You won't get in-person coaching, nor video coaching—everything is done through the chat service, including communications with your personal health coach.

Coaches might not be experts: It's true that all Noom health coaches are approved by the National Consortium for Credentialing Health and Wellness Coaches (NCCHWC) and that Noom's health coach training platform, "Noomiversity," is approved by the National Board for Health & Wellness Coaches (NBHWC). However, that doesn't mean all of their coaches are certified nutritionists, registered dietitians, personal trainers, doctors, or any other credentialed health professional outside of Noom's independent training program.

The color approach may cause problems: While the color-labeling approach to food selection works for some people, for others, it could result in disordered eating habits or an unhealthy relationship with food. For example, almond butter is labeled as a red food because of its high-calorie content, but almond butter is a perfectly healthy food when eaten in moderation.

Is the Noom Diet a Healthy Choice for You?

The Department of Agriculture (USDA) recommends that we fill our plates with a balanced mix of protein, grains, fruits, vegetables, and dairy products for most meals. The Noom diet mostly aligns with these principles, particularly since it recommends limiting the consumption of some "red label" foods that are otherwise considered healthy.

Noom also has a diabetes prevention program that has been officially recognized by the Centers for Disease Control and Prevention (CDC) for its efficacy, a first of its kind for fully mobile-based weight loss programs. The Diabetes Prevention Plan costs $89.99 per month, but it includes more perks than the Healthy Weight Program, such as a specific focus on blood sugar control.

Health Benefits

Despite its relative newness to the wellness scene (Noom was founded in 2009), Noom has quite a body of scientific literature behind it.

Here are the results of some key studies about the Noom program:

• In one 2016 study of more than 35,000 people, researchers found that 77% of Noom users reported losing weight after using the app for nine months.

• Another 2016 study—this one on the National Diabetes Prevention Program—found that the participants all showed significant weight loss after 16 and 24 weeks of using Noom. This study was limited, however, in that it didn't compare Noom to another diabetes diet, so it's hard to make any conclusions about Noom over another diet plan.

• A 2017 study showed that after 12 weeks of using Noom, participants lost an average of

7.5% of their body fat, and after one year, they had maintained a loss of 5.2%.

- This 2017 study shows that Noom's psychological approach is scientifically grounded and can lead to significant weight loss with self-adherence from the participant.

Health Risks

While there are no common health risks associated with the Noom diet, those who have had or are at risk of an eating disorder may want to avoid a weight loss program that requires meticulous tracking of daily food habits and advises against eating some foods that are still considered healthy.

Noom's food guide

Noom recommends eating based on calorie density and categorizes foods as green, yellow, or red accordingly.

The app recommends consuming a set percentage of foods from each color — 30% green, 45% yellow, and 25% red.

According to the Noom website, these are examples of foods for each color (26). They also provide a comprehensive list of foods.

Noom's Food Groups

GreenYellowRed

These foods, which are the least calorie-dense and contain the highest concentration of nutrients, should be what you eat most.

Hearty Veggies: Sweet potatoes, spinach, broccoli

Fruits: apples, strawberries, blueberries

Dairy & Dairy Alternatives: Non-fat cheese, skim milk, unsweetened alternate milks

Whole Grains: Brown rice, oatmeal, whole-grain bread

Beverages: unsweetened tea and coffee

Noom Diet Sample meal plan

Below is an example of one week's meals using recipes from Noom.

This meal plan wouldn't apply to everyone since calorie recommendations are individualized, but it shares a general overview of foods included from the color categories above.

As long as the majority of your diet contains foods in the green and yellow categories, you can include foods categorized as red — such as chocolate cake — in small portions.

Monday

- Breakfast: raspberry yogurt parfait

- Lunch: vegetarian barley soup

- Snack: creamy cucumber and dill salad

- Dinner: fennel, orange, and arugula salad

Tuesday

- Breakfast: banana-ginger smoothie

- Lunch: roasted orange tilapia and asparagus

- Snack: deviled eggs

- Dinner: mushroom and rice soup

Wednesday

- Breakfast: vegetable skillet frittata

- Lunch: broccoli quinoa pilaf

- Snack: homemade yogurt pops

- Dinner: pork lettuce wraps

Thursday

- Breakfast: egg sandwich

- Lunch: chicken and avocado pita pockets

- Snack: mixed nuts

- Dinner: pasta with shellfish and mushrooms

Friday

- Breakfast: spinach-tomato frittata

- Lunch: salmon with tabbouleh salad

- Snack: chocolate cake

- Dinner: grilled chicken with corn salsa

Saturday

- Breakfast: banana-apple and nut oatmeal

- Lunch: turkey cheddar tacos

- Snack: hummus and peppers

- Dinner: green bean casserole

Sunday

- Breakfast: scrambled egg wrap

- Lunch: loaded spinach salad

- Dinner: salmon patties with green beans

- Snack: cream cheese fruit dip with apples

NOOM DIET RECIPES

The following recipes are noom diet-friendly while also being a treat to the taste buds. Try some of these noom diet recipes today.

Noom Green Meal

Preparation time

10 minutes

Ingredients

- 14 oz can bean sprouts drained

- 2 Mini Cucumbers peeled and sliced

- 1/2 Organic Carrot peeled, sliced.

- 3 Stalks of Celery deveined and chopped.

- 1 Serving of Seeds of Change Organic Brown Basmati Rice Cooked

- Navel Orange peeled and divided into chunks

- Garlic Salt Dash

- Optional Items not green

- 1 Tsp Soy Sauce

- 1 Tablespoon Feta Cheese

- 1 Tsp of Trader Joe's Champagne Dressing

Instructions

1. Make sure your shrimp are fully cooked, take off the tail, place in the bowl.

2. Next, add your bean sprouts (drained)

3. Now add the cooked brown basmati rice.

4. Then toss in fresh slices of peeled cucumber.

5. Last, a peeled navel orange.

6. Rinsed and dried large buttercrunch lettuce leaves, plated.

7. As I said, it's a big bowl of yum!

8. Optional items to add in as listed above: Feta, Vinaigrette, and soy sauce.

9. Really add-ins are more a personal choice.

10. If you choose to dress this salad and you don't want any of the aforementioned, consider lemon or lime freshly squeezed atop.

11. Dash with a bit of garlic salt if you like as well.

12. Hold one buttercrunch leaf and then place any of the bowl contents into the lettuce leaf.

13. Roll and enjoy it!

Egg Breakfast Cups

Prepartion time

25 minutes

Ingredients

- 5 eggs

- salt, to taste

- pepper, to taste

MIX AND MATCH FILLINGS

- spinach, chopped

- tomato, diced

- onion, diced fine

- 1 bell pepper, diced fine

- 1 head broccoli, cut into small florets

- parmesan cheese

- cheddar cheese

Instructions

1. Preheat oven to 350°F (180°C).

2. In a measuring cup, beat the eggs until smooth. Set aside.

3. In a greased muffin tin, place your desired combination of fillings into each muffin cup.

4. Season each cup with salt and pepper.

5. Pour the beaten eggs into each muffin cup until the liquid almost reaches the top.

6. Bake for 20 minutes, until set.

7. Enjoy!

Coconut Energy Balls

Prepartion time

1 hour 40 minutes

Ingredients:

- 1 cup unsweetened coconut shreds
- 1/2 cup walnuts
- 1/4 cup pepitas
- 1/2 cup cashews
- 1/4 cup almonds
- 2 tablespoon cacao nibs
- Pinch of sea salt
- Pinch of ground cinnamon (optional to also add ground cardamom)
- 1 teaspoon lemon zest
- 3 drops of stevia extract, to taste (optional)

- 1/2 cup melted coconut oil

- 1/2 cup melted (or warm) coconut butter

- 1/2 cup unsweetened almond milk

- 1/4 cup tahini

Instructions

1. Using a food processor or a high-speed blender, first pulse all the nuts and seeds to a fine flour consistency.

2. Next add in the almond milk, melted coconut oil, coconut butter, stevia, and tahini.

3. Pulse to combine until the mixture resembles dough when you squeeze in between your fingers.

4. Place the mixture in the refrigerator to chill for 20 minutes to harden the mixture just a bit before rolling with your hands.

5. Coconut oil is the binder in the recipe and when chilled, it solidifies, so the heat from your hand may start to soften the mixture.

6. Use your hands to roll the dough into small bite-size balls, place them on a plate or sheet to put in the refrigerator.

7. Repeat until all the dough has been rolled into balls.

8. Immediately chill the coconut energy balls in the fridge for at least 1 hour before serving.

9. Store in the refrigerator for up to 3 weeks in a glass container.

10. Ideally, let thaw for 5 minutes before enjoying.

Deconstructed Grilled Romaine Salad with Cherry Tomatoes, Charred Corn, and Avocado Cream Dressing

Prepartion time

20 minutes

Ingredients

- 2 ears corn, shucked
- 1 head romaine lettuce
- 1 pint cherry tomatoes, sliced in half

For the dressing

- 1 avocado, pitted with skin removed
- 1 tablespoon lime juice
- 1/4 teaspoon salt
- 1/4 cup low-fat plain Greek yogurt
- 3 tablespoons canola or vegetable oil
- 1 garlic clove

Instructions

1. Heat a grill or oven burner to medium-high heat.

2. Place shucked corn directly on the grill or lay flat on the oven burner.

3. Once kernels are evenly charred (but not burnt), turn the ear of corn.

4. Repeat this process until both ears are charred (about 10 to 12 minutes).

5. Set aside to cool.

6. Place lettuce on the grill (or grill pan in the oven) and char the outside (about 1 minute on each side).

7. Set aside to cool.

8. While corn and lettuce cool, make the dressing.

9. Add avocado, lime juice, salt, yogurt, oil, and garlic to a food processor, and blend until smooth.

10. Once the corn is cool enough to touch, cut kernels from the ear.

11. Combine corn with cherry tomatoes and toss with dressing (or dollop dressing on at the end to control the amount).

12. Place corn and tomato mixture on top of the lettuce and enjoy.

Healthy Slow Cooker Lentil and Vegetable Soup

Prepartion time

16 hours 25 minutes

Ingredients

- 1 1/2 cups red lentils

- 4 large carrots peeled and chopped

- 1 red bell pepper chopped

- 2 celery stalks chopped

- 1/2 a bunch of kale about 4 leaves stems removed and chopped

- 2 russet potatoes peeled and chopped

- 1 jalapeno chopped (optional)

- 2 cloves of garlic pressed
- 1/2 an onion chopped
- 1 teaspoon salt
- 1 teaspoon parsley
- 1/2 teaspoon paprika
- 1/2 teaspoon oregano
- 1/2 teaspoon garlic salt
- 1/4 teaspoon cayenne pepper
- 6 1/2 cups vegetable stock

Instructions

1. Place all ingredients in a slow cooker and pour in vegetable stock.

2. Cook on high for 5 hours, or low for 8 hours (low is preferred). Stir a few times throughout the cooking.

3. If you like a more brothy soup, add in 1-2 cups additional stock.

4. Serve with a dollop of sour cream and crusty bread on the side (optional)

Banana-Apple And Nut Oatmeal

Prepartion time

6 minutes

Ingredients

- ¼ cup quick cooking oats

- ½ cup skimmed milk or almond milk
- ¼ tbsp flaxseeds
- ½ medium apple, diced
- 1 tbsp walnuts, chopped
- ½ banana, peeled and sliced
- 1 tbsp honey

Instructions

1. Combine oats, milk, flaxseeds and honey in a microwave-safe bowl.

2. Cook in a microwave for 1½ minutes (you may need to adjust depending on the microwave).

3. Stir the mixture, top with walnuts, apples and bananas. Serve hot.

Chicken And Avocado Pitta Pockets

Prepartion time

5 minutes

Ingredients

- 500g cooked chicken breast, cut into small pieces
- ¼ cup grated reduced-fat cheddar cheese
- ¾ cup diced avocado
- ½ cup bell peppers, seeded and chopped

- ½ cup celery, chopped
- ½ cup cucumber, chopped
- ½ cup carrots, peeled and shredded
- ½ cup cauliflower, finely chopped
- ¼ cup red onion, chopped
- 6tbsp balsamic dressing
- 4 wholewheat pittas, halved

Instructions

1. Toss the chicken, cheddar and vegetables with the dressing.

2. Fill each pitta half with approximately ¾ cup of the mixture.

Turkey Cheddar Tacos

Prepartion time

20 minutes

Ingredients

- 1 cup shredded cooked turkey breast
- 2tbsp drained pickled jalapeño
- 1tbsp fat-free mayonnaise
- 2tbsp fresh chopped coriander
- Zest and juice of 1 lime
- 4 6in/20cm fat-free flour tortillas
- 1 cup shredded lettuce
- 1 cup cherry tomatoes, halved or quartered

- ½ cup grated reduced-fat cheddar cheese

Instructions

1. Combine the turkey, pickled jalapeño, mayonnaise, coriander, lime zest and lime juice in a medium bowl.

2. Warm a large nonstick frying pan over a medium-high heat.

3. Add the tortillas, one at a time, and warm until crisp and dark brown in spots, about one minute on each side.

4. Top each tortilla with ¼ cup of the turkey mixture, spreading it almost to the edge.

5. Top with ¼ cup of lettuce, about ¼ cup of tomatoes and 2tbsp of the cheddar.

Salsa Verde Chicken Tacos

Prepartion time

10 minutes

Ingredients:

- 8 corn tortillas

- 3 cups de-skinned, shredded rotisserie chicken

- 2 cups bottled salsa verde

- 1 cup shredded cheddar cheese or other favorite

- 1 medium onion minced

- 1 cup chopped fresh cilantro

- 2 limes quartered

Instructions

1. Heat tortillas directly on burner or in a saute pan until pliable.

2. Combine chicken and salsa in a large mixing bowl and divide among the tortillas.

3. Top with shredded cheese, minced onion, and cilantro.

4. Serve with lime wedges.

Chinese Chicken Salad

Prepartion time

5 minutes

Ingredients:

- 1 head napa cabbage, cored and sliced into thin strips

- 1 tablespoon agave nectar, sugar, or honey

- 2 cups chopped or shredded chicken (freshly grilled or from a store bought rotisserie chicken)

- 1 cup fresh cilantro leaves

- 1 cup clementine or mandarin oranges

- ¼ cup sliced almonds, toasted

- 1 pinch each of salt and pepper

Instructions

1. Toss cabbage strips in large bowl with the sugar.

2. If you prefer the chicken to be warmed, heat it in the microwave for 30 seconds with a tablespoon of water or balsamic vinegar.

3. Toss all ingredients together in the large bowl and season with salt and pepper.

Spicy Thai Basil Chicken

Prepartion time

7 minutes

Ingredients:

- 1 tablespoon peanut or canola oil
- 1 medium red onion, thinly sliced
- 2 jalapeño peppers, thinly sliced
- 4 cloves garlic, minced
- 1 pound boneless skinless chicken breasts, cut into small pieces
- 2 tablespoon soy sauce and a dash of Worcestershire sauce
- 1 tablespoon sugar
- 1 tablespoon low-sodium soy sauce
- 2 cups fresh basil leaves (Thai basil of available)
- 2 cups rice, cooked

Instructions

1. Heat the oil in a wok or large skillet.

2. When hot, add the onion, jalapeños, and garlic and saute for 2 minutes, stirring to keep the ingredients in motion.

3. Add the chicken and cook for 2 to 3 minutes. The meat will begin to brown.

4. Add the sauces, sugar, and basil.

5. Cook for 1 minute more.

6. Serve over rice.

Chipotle Honey Mustard Chicken Fingers

Prepartion time

20 minutes

Ingredients:

- 1 pound boneless, skinless chicken tenders
- 1 pinch salt and black pepper to taste
- 3 egg whites, lightly beaten
- 2 cups panko gluten-free bread crumbs
- 2 tablespoons Dijon mustard
- 1 teaspoon chipotle spice mix
- 1 tablespoon honey

Instructions

1. Preheat the oven to 450°F.

2. Season the chicken with salt and pepper.

3. Place the egg whites in a shallow bowl.

4. Place the crumbs on a plate and season them with salt and pepper.

5. Dip the chicken tenders into the egg, then toss in the crumbs, being sure to coat fully.

6. Place the breaded chicken pieces on a baking sheet coated with nonstick cooking spray and bake for 10 to 12 minutes, until the crumbs have browned and the chicken is firm.

7. Combine mustard, chipotle spice mix, and honey in a large bowl to make the sauce

8. Toss the cooked chicken tenders in the mixture so they are evenly coated with the spicy-sweet sauce.

Chicken Fajita Burritos

Prepartion time

15 minutes

Ingredients:

- 1/2 tablespoon canola oil

- 1 large onion, sliced

- 1 red bell pepper, sliced

- 1 poblano or green bell pepper, sliced

- 1 pinch salt and black pepper
- 1/2 can black beans, drained
- 1/4 teaspoon cumin
- 1 lime, juiced
- 2 tablespoons hot sauce
- 4 flour tortillas (10")
- 1 cup jack cheese, shredded
- 2 cups shredded chicken (about half a rotisserie chicken)
- 1 cup tomato salsa or salsa verde

Instructions

1. Heat the oil in a large skillet over high heat.

2. Add the onion and all of the peppers.

3. Cook for about seven to eight minutes or until browned.

4. Add salt and pepper.

5. Combine the beans with the cumin in a saucepan.

6. Warm through and keep on low, adding a teaspoon of water here and there to prevent them from drying out.

7. Add the lime juice and a few shakes of hot sauce as well.

8. Preheat a griddle, cast-iron skillet, or large nonstick pan over medium heat.

9. Preheat each tortilla for a few seconds (to make more pliable) before building each burrito.

10. Sprinkle on some cheese, beans, onion-pepper mixture, chicken, and salsa per tortilla.

11. Roll each into a burrito.

12. Place each completed burrito on the skillet.

13. Cook for a minute on each side to toast. Then serve.

Brown Rice Chicken Risotto

Prepartion time

35 minutes

Ingredients

- 2 cups of water.

- 2 tbsp of olive oil.

- 1 of red onion.

- 3 of large carrots.

- 1 large can of diced tomatoes in juice.

- 1 1/4 cups of brown rice

- salt

- pepper.

- 3 of frozen chicken thighs.

Instructions

1. Wash the rice.

2. Chop up the onion and carrots. I tend to use baby carrots because that is what I have in the fridge for my kids. It isn't required that the

chicken is frozen but it is certainly very convenient..

3. Add water, olive oil, the vegetables, rice, salt, and pepper to the Instant Pot and stir.

4. Then place the frozen chicken in the middle on top of the mixture..

5. Cook on high pressure for 25 minutes and then let naturally cool.

6. Pull the chicken, stir, and serve..

Low-Calorie Chicken Tortilla Soup

Prepartion time

1 hour 15 minutes

INGREDIENTS

- 1 tbsp olive oil extra virgin

- 2 large bell peppers any color

- 2 onions small

- 2 cloves garlic minced

- 6 cups chicken broth low sodium

- 4 cups water

- 2 cans Rotel tomatoes with habaneros 10 oz. cans

- 1 can diced green chiles 4 oz can

- 3 tbsp tomato paste

- 2 lbs. cooked chicken breast boiled and shredded OR browned and chopped

- 2 cans cannelloni beans 15 oz. cans (with liquid)
- 3 tsp cumin
- 2 tsp garlic powder
- Salt to taste
- 1 jalapeño pepper thinly sliced, for garnish
- Yellow corn tortillas

INSTRUCTIONS

1. Heat a large pot and add olive oil.

2. Dice bell peppers and onions and saute in the oil on medium heat until soft. Add minced garlic.

3. Add chicken broth, water, Rotel, green chilis, and tomato paste to pot. Stir.

4. Bring to a boil, then reduce heat and simmer for 30 minutes or so.

5. Add cooked chicken breast, cumin, garlic powder, and salt to taste.

6. Using a blender or immersion blender, puree one can of the cannelloni beans. If you don't have a blender, crush the beans using a masher or a fork until smooth.

7. Simmer for 10 minutes, then add the can of whole cannelloni beans, and the pureed/smashed cannelloni beans.

8. While soup is simmering, cut corn tortillas in small strips and spread them out on a cookie sheet.

9. Spray with cooking spray, then sprinkle with cumin and chili powder (or taco seasoning) and

bake at 375 degrees until golden brown and crispy.

10. Serve soup with crisp tortilla strips and fresh jalapeño slices

Banana-Apple & Nut Oatmeal

Prepartion time

5 minutes

Ingredients:

- 1/4 cup quick cooking oats

- 1/2 cup skim or almond milk

- 1/4 tbsp flaxseed

- 1/2 apple, diced

- 1 tbsp chopped walnuts

- 1/2 banana, peeled and sliced

- 1 tbsp honey

Instructions

1. Combine quick oats, milk, flaxseed, and honey in a microwave-safe bowl.

2. Cook in microwave for 2 1/2 minutes, or longer depending on microwave.

3. Stir the mixture, top with walnuts, apples, and bananas. Serve hot.

Mini Ham and Cheese Quinoa Cups

Prepartion time

1 hour

INGREDIENTS

- 2 cups cooked quinoa (about 3/4 cup uncooked)
- 2 eggs
- 2 egg whites
- 1 cup shredded zucchini
- 1 cup shredded sharp cheddar cheese
- 1/2 cup diced ham
- 1/4 cup loosely packed parsley, chopped
- 2 Tablespoons shredded or grated parmesan cheese
- 2 green onions, chopped

- salt & pepper

Instructions

1. Preheat oven to 350 degrees.

2. Combine all ingredients in a large bowl and mix to combine.

3. Liberally spray a mini muffin tin with non-stick spray and spoon mixture to the top of each cup.

4. Bake for 15-20 minutes, or until the edges of the cups are golden brown.

5. Let cool for at least 5 minutes before removing from the mini muffin tin.

6. To freeze: Place baked cups on a baking sheet then freeze until solid and transfer to a freezer bag.

7. Microwave for 20-40 seconds depending on how many you're reheating.

8. For regular-sized muffin tins: Bake for 25-30 minutes (Note: I have not tested full-sized muffins myself, although several readers have left comments saying this works!)

Healthy Breakfast Sandwich

Prepartion time

45 minutes

Ingredients

- 4 eggs
- 4 egg whites
- 1/4 cup minced chives
- 1/4 cup minced parsley
- 4 whole-wheat English muffins
- 4 1/2-inch round slices Canadian bacon
- 1 large beefsteak tomato, sliced into 1/2-inch thick slices

Instructions

1. Crack eggs and egg whites into a bowl and whisk.

2. Add chives and parsley and stir to incorporate.

3. Spray a large nonstick skillet with cooking spray.

4. Ladle 1/4 egg mixture into skillet and cook, omelet style, until eggs are cooked through, about 1 to 2 minutes per side.

5. Slide omelet onto a plate and repeat with remaining eggs; cover with foil to keep warm.

6. In same skillet, heat Canadian bacon until warm, about 1 to 2 minutes per side.

7. Toast English muffin.

8. Fold omelet in to fit English muffin, then place omelet on 1 muffin half.

9. Top with a bacon slice, then tomato, then top with other muffin half.

Apples and Cinnamon Breakfast Quinoa

Prepartion time

17 minutes

Ingredients

- 1 cup dry quinoa (rinsed well)

- 1 1/2 cups water

- 1 tsp cinnamon + more for sprinkling

- 2 tsp vanilla extract

- 1/2 cup unsweetened applesauce

- 1/4 cup golden raisins

- 1 cup warmed fat-free milk for drizzling (non-dairy milk is fine)

- 1 gala apple (peeled and diced)

- 1/4 cup pecans (chopped)

Instructions

1. Combine quinoa, water, cinnamon and vanilla in a small saucepan and bring to a boil.

2. Reduce to a simmer, cover, and let cook for 15 minutes until quinoa can be fluffed with a fork.

3. Divide cooked quinoa between four bowls then stir in apple sauce, raisins, and pour in warmed milk.

4. Top with fresh cut apples and pecans and a dash of cinnamon.

Breakfast Jar Parfait

Prepartion time

5 minutes

Ingredients

Over Night Oatmeal:

- 1/4 cup of Old fashion Oats
- 1/4 Non Fat Milk
- 1/4 tsp of Vanilla Extract
- Dash of Ground Cinnamon
- 1 tsp. chia seeds

The Mix:

- 1/2 Cup of Plain Non Fat Greek Yogurt
- 1/2 cup of diced Strawberries
- 1/2 Blueberries
- 1/2 Tbsp of Peanut Butter
- Sprinkle of Granola

Instructions

1. The night before make your over night Oatmeal

2. Place oatmeal, milk, vanilla, chia seeds and cinnamon in a bowl, stir and leave in the fridge.

3. In the morning, layer in this order: 1/4 cup of yogurt, 1/4 cup of strawberries, 1/4 cup of blueberries, Oatmeal, Peanut Butter, 1/4 cup of yogurt, 1/4 cup of strawberries, 1/4 cup of blueberries

4. Sprinkle with granola!

5. Enjoy!

Green Monster Smoothie

Prepartion time

5 minutes

Ingredients

- 1 cup unsweetened almond milk

- 1 small banana, frozen

- 2 cups baby spinach

- 1 tablespoon chia seeds

- 1 scoop vanilla protein powder

- 8-10 cup ice cubes

Instructions

1. Blend all of the ingredients together in a blender until smooth.

FREEZER BREAKFAST SANDWICHES

Prepartion time

30 minutes

INGREDIENTS:

- 6 large eggs

- Kosher salt and freshly ground black pepper, to taste

- 6 English muffins, split

- 12 slices deli-sliced ham

- 6 slices cheddar cheese

Instructions

1. Preheat oven to 375 degrees. Lightly oil six 10-ounce ramekins or coat with nonstick spray and place onto a baking sheet.

2. Add one egg to each ramekin, beating slightly; season with salt and pepper, to taste. Place into oven and bake until egg whites are cooked through, about 12-14 minutes.

3. Place one egg over the muffin bottom.

4. Top with 2 slices ham and 1 slice cheese, and then cover with another muffin top to create a sandwich.

5. Repeat with remaining English muffins to make 6 sandwiches.

6. Wrap tightly in plastic wrap and place in the freezer.

7. To reheat, remove plastic wrap from the frozen sandwich and wrap in a paper towel.

8. Place into microwave for 1-2 minutes, or until heated through completely.

9. Serve immediately.

Spinach Quiche Cups

Prepartion time

25 minutes

Ingredients

- a little olive oil (for cooking the mushrooms)
- 8 oz package mini-bella mushrooms, chopped
- ¼ cup water
- 10 oz package fresh spinach (about 284 grams)
- 4 eggs 4 eggs (if the yolks are quite small I use 5 eggs)
- 1 cup 1 cup shredded cheese of your choice (I use mozzarella or the Italian Blend)
- 1-2 tablespoons heavy cream or half-and-half (optional)

- salt and pepper, to taste

Instructions

1. Preheat the oven to 375F or 190C.

2. Heat a little oil in a large skillet.

3. Saute the mushrooms until they are soft, about 5-6 minutes. Set Aside.

4. Place the spinach in a deep pan or in the skillet that you used for the mushrooms.

5. Pour in the water.

6. Using medium heat, cook the spinach just until wilted, about 3-4 mins.

7. Use either your hand or a spatula to pack in the spinach.

8. Drain the excess water really well (especially if you decide to use frozen spinach instead).

9. In a large mixing bowl, whisk the eggs until combined.

10. Add the cooked mushrooms, spinach, cheeses and cream (if using) to the eggs.

11. Mix well.

12. Season with salt and pepper to taste.

13. Divide evenly among the 12 muffin cups.

14. The muffin tray was slightly bigger than usual so I only filled about 10 cups.

15. Bake for about 20-23 minutes, or until it's well set and a tester/toothpick inserted in the center comes out clean.

16. Leave in the pan for a few minutes or just until it's cool enough to handle. It was so easy to remove them from the pan! They practically pop-out!

17. Sprinkle with a little more cheese on top, if desired. Hubby enjoys them with rice on the side!

Blueberry Flax Superfood Smoothie

Prepartion time

5 minutes

Ingredients

- 1 cup blueberries, frozen

- 1 Tablespoon flax seed, ground
- Handful of spinach
- 1/4 cup full-fat Greek yogurt, I used vanilla
- 1 cup coconut milk or any kind of milk

Instructions

1. Place all ingredients in a blender or magic bullet.

2. Mix until smooth.

Peanut Butter and Jelly Quinoa Egg Muffins

Prepartion time

35 minutes

Ingredients

- 1 Cup – 1 1/4 Strawberries diced

- 2/3 Cup Unsweetened Vanilla Almond Milk

- Pinch of salt

- 1/3 Cup Quinoa uncooked

- 1/4 Cup Natural Peanut Butter plus additional for drizzling

- 3-4 Tbsp Honey divided *

- 4 Davidson's Safest Choice Egg Whites

- 1 Davidson's Egg Safest Choice Egg

- 1/4 Cup Roasted Peanuts Finely chopped **

Instructions

1. Preheat your oven to 450, line a baking sheet]with parchment paper and generously (very key!) spray a muffin tin with cooking spray.

2. Toss your strawberries with 1/2 Tbsp of the honey and spread onto the parchment lined baking sheet and place into the oven for 10 minutes, until the strawberries release their juices.

3. Once cooked, spoon them into a strainer to strain out any excess juices. Set aside.

4. In a large pot bring the almond milk and a pinch of salt to a boil. Stir the quinoa into the boiling milk.

5. Cover the pot and cook on low heat until most of the milk is absorbed, about 20-25 minutes.

6. Place the peanut butter into a large bowl and microwave for 1 minute, until it melts.

7. Stir in the honey and the cooked quinoa until well mixed.

8. In a separate small bowl, whisk together the egg whites and egg and pour into the quinoa mixture, stirring until the quinoa begins to absorb the egg. Your mixture will be a little bit soupy.

9. Fill 8 of the muffin tins 1/2 of the way full and then divide the cooked strawberries evenly between them, gently stirring around to evenly distribute them.

10. Cover with the remaining quinoa mixture, and sprinkle with the peanuts.

11. Bake until the quinoa appears set and begins to pull away from the sides of the muffin tin, about 20-25 minutes.

12. Let cool in the pan for 10 minutes and then transfer to a cooling rack to finish cooling.

13. Once cooled, drizzle with additional peanut butter and DEVOUR!

NO BAKE ENERGY BITES

Prepartion time

20 minutes

INGREDIENTS

- 1 cup old-fashioned oats

- 2/3 cup toasted shredded coconut (sweetened or unsweetened)

- 1/2 cup creamy peanut butter

- 1/2 cup ground flaxseed

- 1/2 cup semisweet chocolate chips (or vegan chocolate chips)

- 1/3 cup honey

- 1 tablespoon chia seeds (optional)

- 1 teaspoon vanilla extract

INSTRUCTIONS

1. Stir everything together.

2. Stir all ingredients together in a large mixing bowl until thoroughly combined.

3. Chill. Cover the mixing bowl and chill in the refrigerator for 1-2 hours, or until the mixture is chilled. (This will help the mixture stick together more easily.)

4. Roll into balls. Roll into mixture into 1-inch balls.

5. Serve. Then enjoy immediately! Or refrigerate in a sealed container for up to 1 week, or freeze for up to 3 months.

Banana Cookie Overnight Oats

Prepartion time

8 hours 5 minutes

Ingredients

- 1 1/2 Cup Old Fashioned Oats

- 1 1/2 Cup Unsweetened Almond Milk

- 1 Cup Non-Fat Greek Yogurt

- 2 Whole Ripe Bananas

- 1 Teaspoon Cinnamon

- 3 Tablespoons Chia Seeds (Optional if you want a completely Green-Zone Breakfast)

Instructions

1. Mash up the two bananas in a bowl and add all the other ingredients together.

2. Stir well and transfer to a mason jar or a cup with a lid.

3. Place in the refrigerator overnight.

4. In the morning, add any toppings like walnuts, bananas, cinnamon, or blueberries.

Ginger Banana Cookies

Prepartion time

6 hours 40 minutes

Ingredients

- 2 cups all-purpose flour
- 2 ripe bananas, mashed
- 1 cup shortening
- 1 cup coconut sugar
- 1/2 cup salted butter (one stick)
- 2 teaspoons baking powder
- 2 teaspoons grated fresh ginger
- 2 teaspoons ground ginger
- 2 teaspoons banana extract
- 1 teaspoon vanilla extract

- 1 teaspoon cinnamon

- 1/2 teaspoon salt

Instructions

1. In a large mixing bowl, cream together butter and coconut sugar until fluffy.

2. Add eggs, then banana and vanilla flavoring, mixing thoroughly after each ingredient addition.

3. Mash two bananas in a medium-sized bowl.

4. Add bananas and grated ginger root to the wet ingredients; mix thoroughly.

5. In another large mixing bowl, whisk together dry ingredients.

6. Add dry ingredients in small sections to the wet ingredients, mixing thoroughly after each addition.

7. Mix batter until fully combined; it should be wet but thick, not runny.

8. Cover batter in mixing bowl and refrigerate for 5-6 hours or overnight.

9. Once the batter is chilled, preheat the oven to 400º F.

10. Line baking sheets with parchment paper or silicone mats.

11. Using two greased spoons, drop tablespoon-size dollops of batter onto the baking sheets about one-half to one inch apart; the cookies will spread just a bit in the oven.

12. Bake for 10 minutes or until golden brown around the edges.

13. Let cool on baking sheets for 5 minutes before transferring to wire racks to cool completely.

Party Potatoes

Prepartion time

45 minutes

Ingredients

- 8-10 Yukon Gold potatoes

- 8 ounces cream cheese

- 1 cup sour cream

- garlic salt (to taste)
- 1 teaspoon paprika
- milk (as needed)

Instructions

1. Preheat oven to 350?. Wash, peel, and cut potatoes into one-inch cubes.

2. Bring a large pot of water to a boil and cook potatoes until tender (about 15 minutes).

3. Combine softened cream cheese and sour cream into a bowl and mix thoroughly.

4. Drain potatoes, then mash or mix. Slowly add in the cheese mixture and garlic salt.

5. If the mixture seems too thick, add some milk.

6. Transfer to casserole dish and bake uncovered at 350? for 45 minutes.

7. Sprinkle with paprika and enjoy!

PROTEIN-PACKED OMELET

Prepartion time

15 minutes

Ingredients

- ½ cup egg whites

- 2 ounces of cooked shredded chicken

- 1 cup of spinach

Veggies

- Tomato
- Bell pepper
- Onion

Instructions

1. Combine ½ cup egg whites with 2 ounces of cooked shredded chicken.

2. Add 1 cup of spinach and a few handfuls of your favorite veggies (tomato, bell pepper, onion, etc.).

3. Heat in a nonstick skillet until eggs are cooked through.

4. Season with salt and pepper to taste.

Avocado and Egg Lunch

Prepartion time

20 minutes

Ingredients

- 1 Avocado Peeled, sliced into 8 wedges
- 1 Egg poached
- 8 stalks Baby asparagus roasted
- 1 tbsp Balsamic vinegar

- Black pepper fresh ground

Instructions

1. Pre-heat oven to 350° F.

2. Place baby asparagus on small baking sheet, pour a little olive oil over it and shake and roll a bit, to help coat the stalks.

3. Pour a tablespoon of balsamic vinegar over the stalks and roll them in it.

4. Bring a small pot of water to a boil.

5. Next place the asparagus in the oven, for 5 to 7 minutes, taking care to not leave it in too long! Poach the egg for about 3 minutes.

6. While the egg is poaching and asparagus is in the oven, peel and wedge the avocado and place on a plate in spiral form.

7. Place asparagus between wedges of avocado, and plate the poached egg in the center.

8. Garnish with fresh ground black pepper and additional balsamic vinegar if desired.

Peanut Butter and Jelly Cottage Cheese Breakfast Bowl

Prepartion time

5 minutes

Ingredients

- 1/2 cup cottage cheese
- 1/4 cup rolled oats
- 1 Tbsp jam (any flavor)
- 1 Tbsp peanut butter

Instructions

1. Add all the ingredients to a bowl or container.

2. Enjoy immediately or refrigerate in an air-tight container up to four days.

Printed in Great Britain
by Amazon